Table of Contents

INTRODUCTION

Intermittent fasting (IF) is one of the most popular eating patterns among Americans who follow a diet or eating pattern. IF doesn't restrict what you can eat, only when you can eat. Some studies have shown that IF can help manage weight, reduce blood pressure, and lower cholesterol, but the evidence of long-term benefits is limited. Intermittent fasting (IF) remains one of the most popular eating patterns among Americans following a diet plan, even though its long-term benefits are still unknown.

It's a method of calorie restriction based on timing. Unlike other eating patterns, IF is based on when you eat, not what you eat.This eating pattern has become more mainstream as many celebrities and influencers swear by it. The research on IF is mixed. A new study showed that time-restricted eating may help people with obesity lose weight,1 while another found that intermittent fasting had no significant impact on weight loss. Most of the other existing studies that support this eating pattern were conducted on animals, while the few studies involving humans have been short and often include a small sample size.

INTERMITTENT FASTING PLANS

Although the research on IF is mixed, some people still follow a schedule to support their weight loss goals or to maintain their fitness level. There are three main IF schedules:

Alternate-day Fasting: Rotate between days of eating and days of fasting. On fasting days, you're not allowed to consume any calories aside from water, black coffee, or tea. On non-fasting days, you can eat anything you want.

Modified Fasting: There are different approaches to this, such as fasting two days a week (called the 5:2 fast) and eating normally for the other five days, restricting calories to a certain percentage of your normal intake on fasting days, or restricting calories to a certain number (e.g., 500 calories) on fasting days.

Time-restricted Fasting: This means fasting for a set number of hours, which can vary from eight to 12 hours a day. Many people try to include sleep time in their fast to make this more manageable.

Is Intermittent Fasting Safe?

For most healthy adults, time-restricted eating is safe. IF can help people "become more cognizant of a healthy eating pattern," but they do have to be cautious about how they practice it. Although IF doesn't restrict food choices, it's still important to consider your overall diet quality. "If you don't change your food choices, it's really not going to make any difference," Smalling said. People with certain conditions, such as diabetes, should consider talking to a trusted healthcare provider before trying out IF, she added. For people who use insulin, fasting might lead to hypoglycemia, a condition that occurs when blood sugar level drops too low.

According to Susie, IF is not recommended for children or people who are pregnant or breastfeeding. Some experts are also cautious about alternate-day and modified fasting schedules because these plans could lead to decreased concentration, low energy levels, or hunger pains. For now,

Smalling said, a lot more long-term research needs to be done to confirm the benefits of this eating pattern.

What This Means For You

If you have a history of disordered eating, IF may not be the right eating plan for you. Speak with a healthcare provider to evaluate your health history before getting on an IF schedule.

How to Time Meals While Intermittent Fasting for Diabetes

Intermittent fasting (IF) for people with diabetes has the potential benefit of improving blood glucose—and possibly reversing diabetes or going into "remission." The key is balancing these benefits with the safety concerns of following this eating plan when taking diabetes medications. IF is a type of eating plan that involves limiting the time period when you eat. There are several different ways to do that, including:

Restricting eating during a certain time of day

Limiting the number of calories during a fasting period

Rotating between normal eating days and fasting days

HISTORY OF DIABETES AND INTERMITTENT FASTING

Fasting has been around for a long time: It has been a historical part of some spiritual traditions stretching back centuries. More recently, IF has been used as part of a healthy diet for weight loss, as a "detoxifying" strategy, and more. There's been some debate about whether fasting is healthy for those with diabetes. A growing body of evidence suggests that some IF diets could benefit people with diabetes. Scientists note that when a person fasts may be just as important as the diet itself.

Glucose Metabolism

To understand the benefits of intermittent fasting and diabetes, it's important to know a little about how your body processes glucose and insulin. Insulin is a hormone that enables glucose (sugar) to enter muscle, fat, and liver cells, where it's used for energy. Normally, when blood glucose rises, the pancreas releases insulin. Insulin lowers blood sugar by "unlocking" cells so that they absorb sugar from the bloodstream. That's how your body keeps blood sugar at a healthy level (between 70 to 99 milligrams/deciliter).

Insulin Resistance

Sometimes muscle, fat, and liver cells don't respond normally to insulin. Glucose builds up in the blood because it can't enter the cells. This is called insulin resistance because the cells resist the effects of insulin.bThe pancreas responds by making more insulin. The extra insulin may keep the blood sugar level in a healthy range—until the pancreas can no longer make enough insulin to overcome the insulin resistance of the cells.

Prediabetes

Prediabetes means your blood glucose levels are higher than normal, but not high enough to qualify as diabetes. You may have prediabetes if you have insulin resistance. Prediabetes can also happen if your pancreas doesn't make enough insulin to keep your blood sugar within the normal range. Over time, prediabetes often progresses into type 2 diabetes. Some people have reversed type 2 diabetes after losing 30 pounds or more.3 Although not everyone who loses this much weight will be able to put their diabetes into remission, there are many health benefits to losing weight.

How Intermittent Fasting Works

The primary goal of intermittent fasting for weight loss is to get insulin levels low enough so your body burns stored fat (instead of sugar) for energy.

Here is how it works: When your body breaks down the food you eat, it ends up as molecules in your bloodstream. One such molecule is glucose. It comes from the breakdown of carbohydrates. Your body makes insulin so your cells can store and use that glucose. If you have more blood glucose than your body can use, it gets stored as fat for future use.   When you're not eating meals or snacks, insulin levels drop. When insulin levels are low, fat cells release some of the stored fat so it can be used for energy. That results in weight loss.

Benefits of Intermittent Fasting
A few small studies have shown that intermittent fasting can have health benefits for people with diabetes, including:

Weight loss

Lowering insulin requirements

A long-term study published in the New England Journal of Medicine showed that fasting can:

Lessen inflammation

Lower insulin levels

Improve a wide range of illnesses such as asthma, arthritis, and more

Detox the body

Help the body rid itself of damaged cells, which may lower the risk of cancer

Other reported benefits of fasting include:

Lower triglycerides and LDL ("bad") cholesterol levels

Lower blood pressure

Side Effects

Intermittent fasting is safe for most people, but it isn't right for everyone. IF diets may not be safe for people who are pregnant or breastfeeding, under age 18, have a history of eating disorders, or have diabetes.8 Fasting does have some downsides. Side effects of IF diets can include:

Bad breath (which often results from low-carb diets)

Trouble concentrating

Excessive hunger

Irritability

Insomnia

Headaches

Dehydration

Daytime sleepiness

Low energy levels that may impact your ability to exercise, which is important for people with diabetes

A much higher risk of low blood sugar (hypoglycemia)

High blood sugar (hyperglycemia), if the liver responds to fasting by releasing stored glucose9

More research is needed to understand how common and how severe these side effects could be. Check with your healthcare provider before making major changes to your diet if you have diabetes. Some side effects, like hyperglycemia or hypoglycemia, could be dangerous for people with diabetes. Talk to your healthcare provider before you start any type of IF diet.5

Types of IF Diets for Diabetes

Several IF diets have proven safe and effective for people with diabetes. Here's a look at the research.

The 5:2 Diet

The popular 5:2 diet was introduced in Dr. Jason Fung's best-selling book "The Obesity Code" in 2016.4 It involves eating a recommended amount of calories five days per week, with two non-consecutive days of eating a reduced-calorie diet. On fasting days, you don't stop eating altogether—you just reduce the number of calories. If you have diabetes and want to try the 5:2 diet, speak to your healthcare provider or diabetes team. They'll help you set a target calorie intake for the fasting and non-fasting days. Studies have shown that the 5:2 diet may lower insulin resistance. It may also help with weight loss in people with type 2 diabetes or prediabetes. The first long-term study of the 5:2 diet was published in 2018 by the Journal of the American Medical Association (JAMA). It found that fasting could be effective for those with diabetes who have trouble sticking to a long-term, daily diet regimen. The study tracked 137 people with type 2 diabetes:

Half of them followed the 5:2 diet. They fasted for two non-consecutive days per week, taking in 500 to 600 calories on the fasting days. They ate normally on the other five days.

The other half ate a daily restricted diet of 1200 to 1500 calories per day.

The study found that those who followed the 5:2 diet were just as likely to control their blood sugar levels as those on the daily restricted-calorie diet. Researchers said the 5:2

diet "may be superior to continuous energy restriction for weight reduction."

Some experts question the safety of the 5:2 diet for people with diabetes. However, a long-term study published in 2018 reported that "fasting is safe for those with diet-controlled type 2 diabetes."

The study authors concluded that those who take insulin or oral diabetes medications such as glyburide or metformin need very close monitoring. They may need to adjust their dosages. This is because fasting can cause hypoglycemia if you're taking medications that lower your blood sugar. This study found the 5:2 diet safe for those with diabetes. Still, it's important to talk to your healthcare provider before fasting or starting any other type of diet.

Early Time-Restricted Feeding Diet (eTRF)

With an early time-restricted feeding (eTRF) diet, you fit all your meals into a specific period of time each day. The eTRF diet plan may be an eight-hour, 10-hour, or even a six-hour plan. On the eight-hour plan, if you begin eating at 7:00 a.m., the last meal or snack for the day would be at 3:00 p.m. An example of the 12-hour early time-restricted feeding plan would be when you eat the first meal of the day at 7:00 a.m. and the last meal or snack no later than 7:00 p.m.

How the eTRF Diet Works
The eTRF diet may work with your circadian rhythm. This is the body's internal clock, which controls the timing of sleep, waking, and metabolism. That's why some think the diet could aid weight loss. If you stop eating earlier in the evening, you will extend your overnight fast. According to a study published in the New England Journal of Medicine, fasting triggers some important cell functions, such as lowering blood sugar and boosting metabolism.

Benefits of the eTRF

Benefits of the eTRF diet include:

Less appetite

Weight loss

More fat loss via oxidation (burning of fat)

Lower blood pressure

Study on the eTRF Diet for Diabetes

In a 2018 study, the eight-hour eTRF diet was compared with the 12-hour diet. The study found that the eight-hour group had dramatically lower insulin levels than the 12-hour group. Both groups maintained their weight. And both groups lowered insulin and blood pressure.

Safe Ways to Do Intermittent Fasting With Diabetes

Follow these tips if you have diabetes and plan to start an IF diet:

Consult with your diabetes team about whether the diet is a good choice for you. Follow their advice on any changes to your medication schedule. You want to be sure to keep a healthy blood glucose level.

Test your blood glucose levels often.

If you have symptoms of hypoglycemia, break the fast immediately. Use your action plan, such as taking glucose tablets followed by a snack. Talk to your healthcare provider before resuming the fast.

If you have type 1 diabetes, watch for signs of hyperglycemia when you fast. These include fatigue, extreme thirst, and frequent urination. Contact your healthcare provider right away if you have these symptoms or your blood sugar level stays high.

Meal Planning Tips

As with any eating plan, it's important to maintain a balanced diet to ensure your body is getting the nutrition it needs for long-term health. Include these meal-planning tips in your IF plan:

Include foods from all of the food groups to get adequate fiber, protein, vitamins, and minerals.

Eat foods that fill you up and keep your blood sugar steady during the fast, such as lean protein (fish, seafood, poultry), beans, nuts, fruits, vegetables, and fresh salads.

Don't overeat during the non-fasting periods.

Just before you fast, eat foods that are more slowly absorbed, including foods that are lower on the glycemic index scale: carrots, dark leafy greens, non-starchy vegetables, most fruits, beans, oatmeal, bran cereals, quinoa, barley, nuts, milk, and yogurt.14 These foods are often high in fiber or protein and are digested slowly.

When you break the fast, limit the amount of fatty and sugary foods you eat. Instead of frying, try grilling or baking chicken or fish; choose fresh fruit instead of ice cream, bakery items, and candy.

Drink lots of fluids (mostly water) during the fast to avoid dehydration. Avoid sugary drinks.

The safety of fasting for those with type 1 diabetes has not been fully established. If you have type 1 diabetes, you should never fast without first discussing it with your healthcare provider.

How Long to Fast Before Blood Work

You may have to fast—avoiding anything but water—for eight to 12 hours before a blood test. This is because nutrients from foods and beverages are absorbed into your blood, which can cause inaccurate results. Make sure you are clear about whether or not you need to fast for the test(s) you are scheduled for so you can avoid having to repeat them.

Tests That Require Fasting

Most blood tests actually do not require fasting, but some common ones do. These include:

Basic metabolic panel

Blood glucose test

Cholesterol test

Triglyceride level test

Lipoprotein panel

High-density lipoprotein (HDL) level test

Low-density lipoprotein (LDL) level test

Renal function panel

Liver function tests

Iron level test

Most lab tests drawn in pregnancy do not require fasting, with the exception of the glucose challenge test. This test is performed to screen for a condition called gestational diabetes. For this test, you will be asked to consume a special sugary beverage that contains a specific amount of glucose. Your blood glucose level will be tested at specific time intervals.

How Long You Need to Fast

Generally, you should fast for eight to 12 hours before lab work that requires it. You can always clarify how long to fast with your healthcare provider. If you are unsure, aim for 12 hours of fasting. For example, if you schedule your test for first thing in the morning, you should generally not eat anything after dinnertime the night before.

Why Do You Need to Fast?

Everything you eat or drink is broken down by your digestive system and absorbed into your bloodstream. The nutrients from foods and beverages circulate the body for a period of time so they can be "delivered" throughout the body. This can take hours, which is why you may be asked to fast for a period of time before certain blood tests. For laboratory tests that don't examine the levels of certain nutrients or other substances in your blood, eating and drinking should not affect the results. For those that do, however, anything you eat or drink in the hours prior may produce an inaccurate result.

For example, eating before a blood glucose test will raise your blood sugar and lead to inaccurate test results, so fasting is required. However, the hemoglobin A1c test—also done for diabetes—does not require fasting. This is because it looks at a marker of blood sugar control over the past few months, rather than directly measuring blood sugar. An inaccurate test result is problematic for several reasons:

It may cause you unnecessary stress if your results are outside the range of normal.

It may prompt your healthcare provider to alter a medication dose.

It may prompt additional testing that is unnecessary and costly.

It may be compared to results from previous tests in which you did fast.

How to Fast for Blood Work

Your healthcare provider will give you details on how long you need to fast before your blood test. Most of these types of tests are scheduled for first thing in the morning, so you can sleep during the fasting period. During the fasting period, you should avoid all drinks (including coffee and tea) except for water. Drinking water is even encouraged before blood work because a 12-hour fast from drinking fluids can make you slightly dehydrated. This causes your veins to flatten and makes them harder to find for a venipuncture. Your healthcare provider may also ask you to avoid chewing gum and smoking. In some cases, you may also have to abstain from exercising.

What Does NPO After Midnight Mean?

"NPO after midnight" means "nil per os," which is Latin for "nothing by mouth"—including water. This is used before procedures and is not the same type of fasting required for blood work.

Medication and Blood Tests

Even if you are asked to fast for blood work, you should take your prescribed medications with water, unless specifically requested not to do so. The exception to this is vitamins and supplements. These may affect certain lab tests, so they should be held the morning of a lab test. Discuss what medications you are taking with your healthcare provider and clarify ahead of time if you have any questions on holding medications before blood work.

What to Do If You Accidentally Eat or Drink

If you accidentally ate or drank before your test, let your healthcare provider know. Depending on the reason the test was ordered, you may be able to go ahead and have your blood drawn. The healthcare provider will just take this into account when interpreting your results. For example, if you are having a screening cholesterol panel and you ate breakfast before the test, it's not necessary to reschedule it. In fact, newer recommendations from the National Lipidology Association state that fasting for a screening lipid panel is optional.

While your breakfast will affect the triglyceride level, other important parts of the test, such as the total cholesterol and HDL (high-density lipoprotein, known as "good" cholesterol) will not be affected. LDL will only be affected if the triglyceride level is very elevated. If the triglyceride level is elevated, you may be asked to come back to repeat the test. On the other hand, if a test was ordered specifically for blood sugar and you ate breakfast, the test may not be useful. Pregnant people who do not fast before undergoing the glucose challenge will be asked to reschedule the test.

Many lab tests do not require fasting. But for those that do, such as blood glucose tests, eating food can affect the results. Check with the healthcare provider who ordered the blood work to see if fasting is necessary, and if so, do not eat for to eight to 12 hours before the test. It's fine to take your prescribed medication and drink water before the test to stay hydrated.

How long does it take to get blood test results?
Depending on the test and how urgently your healthcare provider has indicated on the lab order form, blood test results can come back as soon as under an hour to several days. When the test is marked as "stat," it indicates to the

lab that the test should be run and reported back as soon as possible, whereas "routine" means there is no rush for a result. The timing also depends on whether the test has to be transported to a special lab.

Why would I need to repeat a blood test?

Your healthcare provider may ask that you have a repeat blood test when the results are invalid, to confirm unexpected results, or if not enough blood was provided to run all of the necessary tests. Blood is drawn in special tubes and transported to a lab for testing. The lab equipment requires a certain amount of blood to run the tests. Some lab tests are affected if the blood has sat in the tube for too long, if the tube was not maintained at the proper temperature, or if the blood underwent breakage (hemolysis) during the blood draw.

How do you book a blood test?

Most blood tests require an order from a healthcare provider, such as a physician, nurse practitioner, or physician's assistant. Your healthcare provider's office may have a phlebotomist who can draw the labs right in the office, or you may be asked to go to a separate lab facility. Some facilities take walk-ins, while others require appointments.

When can I eat normally after a blood test?

You can go back to eating and drinking as you normally would once your blood has been drawn. You may want to bring a snack along with you so you can have something to eat as soon as you are done with your appointment.

INTERMITTENT FASTING – DIET PLAN, BENEFITS, AND WEIGHT LOSS

There are several studies that have demonstrated the powerful effects that occur on the brain and body due to intermittent fasting. Some studies have even shown that IF can help you live longer. The following information is your beginner's guide to intermittent fasting.

What is Intermittent Fasting?

This is an eating pattern that cycles through periods of eating and fasting. The Intermittent Fasting plan doesn't specify exact foods that you need to eat, but when you ought to eat them. On this plan, a whole food, nutritious eating regimen is recommended. Hence IF is not a conventional diet, but an eating pattern or habit. In this method, fasting occurs for either 16 hours a day or 24 hours, two times per week. Fasting is not an unfamiliar practice in human evolution. In fact, it is more commonplace than we know. Our ancient hunter and gatherer humans didn't have refrigerators, year-round foods or supermarkets. Sometimes they couldn't find food to eat. In response to this scenario, they learned to function without food for lengthy periods of time.

In modern society, we see fasting occurring for spiritual or religious reasons. For instance, regular fasting is a common practice in many world religions such as Hinduism, Buddhism, Islam, and Judaism. In fact, when you think about it, periodic fasting is more natural than consuming 3 or more meals every single day.

Intermittent Fasting Methods

There are several ways to perform intermittent fasting. The most popular methods are:

16-8 Method

This is also called the Leangains protocol. To follow, you will skip breakfast and restrict your eating period to 8 hours.bFor example, you may eat between 1 to 9 pm but then you will fast for the remaining 16 hours.

5:2 Diet

In this method, you normally eat for five days and restrict your calorie intake to 500 to 600 calories on two non-successive days in the week, i.e. Tuesday and Thursday.

Eat-Stop-Eat

On this plan, you will fast for 24 hours, either once or twice a week. Then eat regularly on non-fasting days. On intermittent fasting, you're reducing your calorie intake which leads to weight loss. However, it will only work if you're not overindulging on junk food or compensating by eating more during allowed eating periods. Most people prefer the 16-8 method because it's more sustainable, simple, and easy to follow. It's no wonder that it's also the most popular!

Is Intermittent Fasting Good for Health?

To determine the answer to this question, let's examine what occurs at the cellular and hormonal levels when you fast intermittently. Many things happen at the molecular and cellular level when you fast. For instance, your body begins to adjust its hormone levels so that it can make all stored body fat more easily accessible. Then your cells initiate vital repair processes and alter gene expression. Here are a few changes that are occurring while you're fasting:

The levels of the Human Growth Hormone (HGH) skyrocket; sometimes increasing as much as 5 times. This benefits muscle gain, and fat loss.

Your insulin sensitivity will improve. By fasting, your insulin levels will drop significantly, which helps make stored body fat easy to access.

When you fast, your cells trigger cellular repair. Autophagy is an example of cell repair. In this process, old cells are removed and digested, including dysfunctional proteins that have accumulated inside.

Intermittent fasting contributes to changes in gene expression which promotes longevity and protection against many diseases.

These changes that occur at the cell, hormone, and gene expression levels all contribute to the many health benefits of this fasting method.

Is Intermittent Fasting Good for Weight loss?
Most people attempt intermittent fasting because of the weight loss that occurs when you follow this plan. By eating fewer meals, intermittent fasting leads to a reduction in caloric intake. This directly affects hormone and insulin levels which aid weight loss. In addition, fasting also helps

trigger the release of norepinephrine; a fat-burning hormone. Even if you fast for a short period, your metabolic rate jumps up by 3.6 to 14%. By eating fewer calories, and burning more calories, you're effectively changing the calorie equation and promoting weight loss.

Many studies have demonstrated that intermittent fasting is an effective weight loss tool. According to a 2014 study conducted at the University of Illinois at Chicago, intermittent fasting caused up to 8% of weight loss over a 24-week period. This is a notable amount of weight loss compared to other methods. This same study found that people following intermittent fasting were able to lose up to 7% of waist and belly fat, which is a known contributor to diseases. The participants in this study were losing approximately 0.55 pounds each week. It is also important to exercise along with IF, this has been proven to help with fat loss and muscle gain. So in a nutshell, intermittent fasting can and will help you lose weight provided you don't compensate by over-eating during the allowable periods. In addition to weight loss, there are significant benefits to metabolic health and the prevention of chronic diseases.

BENEFITS OF INTERMITTENT FASTING FOR HEALTHY LIFE

The benefits of intermittent fasting have been demonstrated in both human and animal studies. There are powerful positive effects on weight control and brain and body health as well. In addition, did you know that intermittent fasting can also help you live a longer life? Listed below, are just a handful of health benefits from intermittent fasting:

1. Insulin Resistance

Intermittent Fasting reduces insulin resistance and helps lower blood sugar levels by up to 6%. Fasting insulin levels are reduced by up to 31%. This provides significant protection from type 2 diabetes. According to this research, it may be considered an auxiliary treatment to prevent the occurrence and development of chronic diseases related to blood sugar and lipids in patients with metabolic syndromes.

2. Anti-Aging

Gaps between eating boost metabolism, inducing our bodies to break down nutrients and burn calories more efficiently. It also affects DNA repair positively and slows down its degradation thus working as an anti-ageing tool. Research indicates that intermittent fasting also increases the levels of antioxidants that fight against the free radicals which cause cell damage and lead to various health issues and skin conditions linked to ageing.

3. Brain Health

When you fast, BDNF hormones increase in the brain. This promotes the growth of new neurons and also provides protection against Alzheimer's disease. Studies show that intermittent fasting increases neuroplasticity in the brain. It optimizes brain functions and increases its resistance to injuries.

4. Heart Health

It has been proven by research that fasting helps reduce LDL cholesterol, blood sugar, inflammatory markers, insulin resistance, and blood triglycerides; all risk factors that contribute to heart disease.

5. Inflammation

Inflammation in the body is caused by cells called monocytes. Studies have shown that fasting contributes to a reduction in the release of these inflammation markers which are a key cause of several chronic diseases.

6. Weight Loss

Perhaps the most noticeable benefit of all, on intermittent fasting you will lose belly fat and visceral fat.

INTERMITTENT FASTING DIET PLAN – WHAT TO EAT AND WHAT TO AVOID

When we opt for intermittent fasting, it takes some time for our bodies to adjust to the new schedule. Over time, it adapts to the changes and realigns its functioning. The food we consume during our eating hours is systematically broken down over the expanse of fasting hours to meet the energy requirements of the body. Thus, it's crucial to be conscious of what we eat, how much of it is required by our body and how it affects our system.

For example, if we consume too many calories, they will be stored in our body as fat but a calorie deficit will make you feel fatigued and nauseous. To ensure that you get the most out of intermittent fasting, it's vital to consume nutritious foods and beverages during the eating periods. Although there is no water-tight diet plan, including some foods and avoiding a few others will ensure your goal is achieved in the healthiest way possible.

Foods To Eat During Intermittent Fasting

Unsweetened Beverage

Keeping your body hydrated is of paramount importance when it comes to fasting. A lot of people assume that they are not supposed to have even liquids during intermittent fasting but that's not the case. Have as much water as possible. You can also go ahead and enjoy your cup of herbal tea or black coffee. However, remember not to mix sugar as it counts as calorie intake and will break your fast. You can also savour coconut water, buttermilk, black coffee and fresh lemon water (without sugar) during your hours of fasting. These drinks will also keep your hunger pangs at bay.

Fruits

It goes without saying that fruits are the go-to food item during fasting. However, there are a few fruits that stand above others when it comes to their nutritional value. For example, avocados, which are rich in unsaturated fat, should be your first choice during intermittent fasting. Research suggests that unsaturated fat keeps you fuller for longer. Another great option is berries. They are a great source of flavonoids and thus help regulate cellular activities in our body during the fasting hours when our bodies are susceptible to oxidative damage. Furthermore, choosing fruits that are low in fructose (fruit sugar) promotes better metabolism without increasing your calorie intake.

Vegetables

Vegetables are another obvious addition to this list. You may consume all types of vegetables during your eating hours. Cruciferous vegetables like cauliflower, broccoli, Brussel sprouts etc. in particular should be a part of your diet during intermittent fasting. According to studies, these fibre-rich vegetables ensure you feel fuller for longer. Additionally, they add bulk to your stool and ensure a smooth bowel movement even when your food intake is restricted to only a few hours.

Whole Grains

Packed with both protein and fibre, whole grains are your best friends during intermittent fasting. They keep you full for longer, ensure your energy requirements are met and keep your digestive system healthy even while you switch between eating and fasting. Opt for food items made from whole grains such as buckwheat, barley, quinoa, oats, brown rice, etc.

Lean Protein

Lean protein foods like paneer, egg whites, skinless chicken, fish, etc. are also rich in vitamin B. Vitamin B regulates energy levels, supports brain functions and induces proper metabolism. It also assists in healthy digestion. Protein takes longer to break down and thus curbs cravings. Consuming lean proteins replenishes the essential vitamins and minerals needed to keep your metabolism running efficiently.

Legumes

We often hear our parents and adults saying that legumes like beans and lentils are good for health but did you know they can go a long way during intermittent fasting? Their negligible fat and cholesterol content along with high protein and folates like zinc magnesium and iron make them a tough contender against meat protein. Being high in protein and fibre, keep your hunger at bay and your calorie count under check.

Foods To Avoid During Intermittent Fasting

Processed Food

Processed foods of any kind should be off your list if you're on an intermittent fasting routine. It has been subjected to a heavy manufacturing process where it loses its health benefits and is packed with empty calories.

Research suggests that heavily processed foods cause overeating and subsequent weight gain. Choose healthier options like whole wheat flour or healthy grains instead of refined flour and refined grains.

Sugary Products

Sugar is broken down very quickly by our systems. This not only causes a spike in blood sugar but even leaves us feeling hungry in a very short span of time. Furthermore, sugar doesn't contain any minerals and nutrients but only adds to the calorie count. Thus, it's advisable to abstain from having food high in sugar.

Junk Food/ Convenience Food

You must realise that with every bite you take of junk food you're missing out on nutrients that you could have otherwise consumed. As mentioned above, our bodies utilise the energy from the food we consume to keep our system functioning smoothly during hours of fasting. Make mindful decisions about what you put on your plate. Not just while you're fasting but life in general.

12 BURNING QUESTIONS ABOUT INTERMITTENT FASTING, ANSWERED

Forget counting calories or swearing off carbs — the latest diet fad doesn't put limitations on what you eat. Rather, it focuses on when. This way of eating is called intermittent fasting (IF), and in the past several years it has risen through the ranks of popular diets, until it's now one of the most-looked-up diets on Google, with hundreds of thousands of searches on average each month. What's the reason for its popularity? "It seems a lot easier for some people. Traditional lifestyle changes tend to rely a lot on calorie counting or point watching or rules, and for some people — especially people with busy lives or who feel pulled in a lot of directions — that feels like a lot of work and effort. So for this, where they literally have to do nothing but skip a meal, it's just a lot easier for them to maintain," says Elizabeth Lowden, MD, a physician in Warrenville, Illinois, who is board certified in obesity medicine, endocrinology, diabetes, and metabolism, and internal medicine. Here, we explore the ins and outs of IF and answer all the questions you're probably asking.

1. What Is Intermittent Fasting, and How Is the Diet Different From Starvation?

IF is a way of eating that calls for alternating between fasting (or significant reduction of calorie intake) and eating at specific times, according to Johns Hopkins Medicine. It's different from other diets in that it's not about eating specific foods. IF is not about depriving yourself, either. Rather, it's about eating your meals during a certain time frame and fasting for the rest of the day and night.

2. What Is the History of Intermittent Fasting (and Fasting in General)?

Fasting has been around since ancient times and has predominantly been practiced within religions, according to a study published in the Journal of the Academy of Nutrition and Dietetics. But the version of IF that's talked about today arose in the past decade or so. According to Harvard Health, IF became more popular around 2012 when the documentary Eat, Fast, and Live Longer aired. The Journal of the Academy of Nutrition and Dietetics study says many books on the topic were published around that time as well, including 2013's The Fast Diet, which added to the buzz. Research followed. "Over the past five years, rigorous research has shown the remarkable benefits of intermittent fasting, which is behind this sudden interest," says Sara Gottfried, MD, the Berkeley, California–based author of Brain Body Diet.

3. How Does Intermittent Fasting Work?

There are a few different versions of IF (outlined below), but each follows the basic premise of certain periods of time during the week (or day) meant for eating and for when food is limited (or avoided entirely), according to Harvard Health.

4. What Are the Different Types of Intermittent Fasting??

The following are the most popular.

16:8

This method calls for 16 hours of fasting and 8 hours of eating during the day. Followers of this method usually skip breakfast and eat between the hours of 11 a.m. and 7 p.m. or noon and 8 p.m. The rest of the night and morning is spent fasting. Dr. Lowden says this approach is commonly referred to as "time-restricted eating."

Alternate-Day Fasting

This involves limiting your calories on fasting days and eating normally on other days. For instance, you might severely restrict calories on Monday, Wednesday, and Friday, and then eat normally on the other days. There are various calorie limits for fasting days, with some calling for 0 calories and others allowing up to 600 calories per day, according to a review published in December 2021 in JAMA Network Open.

5:2 Fasting

A very low number of calories (around 400 to 500) is allowed on the two nonconsecutive "fasting" days of the week. The five other days have no eating restrictions, per Harvard T.H. Chan School of Public Health.

5. Can Intermittent Fasting Help You Lose Weight?

The short answer: probably. "IF gets a lot of press as a weight loss tool, and I recommend it in my practice for weight loss and weight management," Dr. Gottfried says. It's linked to weight loss because significant stretches of time between meals force the body to use the fat stored in cells for energy, according to Harvard Health. Insulin levels decline through this process as the body burns fat. Lowden believes that any weight loss really comes down to calorie restriction. "Overall, people tend to consume fewer calories in a smaller window of time compared with eating all day, and that's what leads to weight loss," she says. A study published in June 2018 in Nutrition and Healthy Aging involving 23 obese adults found that study participants took in about 300 fewer calories per day when participating in the 16:8 approach to IF. The National Institute on Aging notes that IF may work because there's less time for eating, so you naturally take in fewer calories each day.

Versions of IF that restrict eating after a certain time, say 7 p.m., also eliminate nighttime eating, which has been shown to contribute to metabolic syndrome and obesity, according to a study published in December 2018 in BMC Public Health. Some critics, however, say the amount of weight loss to expect from IF isn't any more significant than what you'd see with other calorie-restrictive diets. A study published in the American Journal of Clinical Nutrition in November 2018 found that a diet that cut calories by 20 percent resulted in a similar amount of weight loss to the 5:2 version of IF after one year. Still, IF may be a good option if you find it easier to stick to than other diets.

6. What Are the Touted Benefits of Intermittent Fasting, and Are They Legit?

Here are some of the proposed benefits of IF.

Boosted Weight Loss

A review published in Current Obesity Reports in June 2018 found that most research on IF has supported its link to weight loss, and the data suggest that it can result in between a 5 and 9.9 percent loss of body weight. The 2018 study published in Nutrition and Healthy Aging suggested that alternate-day fasting may produce greater weight loss than time-restricted eating, but that alternate-day fasting may be harder to stick with than time-restricted eating. Ultimately, more research is needed on whether IF can result in sustainable weight loss.

A Lengthened Life

A study published in March 2020 in Cell used a lab model to analyze markers of cell aging, and suggested calorie restriction may slow the aging process by reducing inflammation in the body. Nonetheless, the study is preliminary; the same findings haven't been shown in humans.

Reduced Insulin Resistance

This condition is the hallmark of type 2 diabetes, and overweight increases the likelihood of insulin resistance, according to the Centers for Disease Control and Prevention (CDC). IF can help with insulin resistance by reducing the number of calories consumed overall, per a study published in Nutrients in April 2019.

Improved Heart Health

A study published in Nutrition Journal found that IF helped study participants lose weight, lose fat, and lower their cholesterol levels, leading researchers to conclude eating this way may help people lower their risk of coronary artery disease.

Healthier Metabolic Markers

"What we do know is a lot of those metabolic parameters respond to weight loss in general," Lowden says. "No matter how you lose the weight, you'll have decreased visceral (belly) fat, decreased fasting blood sugars, decreased triglycerides, blood sugar, all those things." Lowden says this has been shown in a few animal studies, but "a lot of the things you'd physiologically expect from a longer fast time aren't necessarily panning out in population studies," she says.

Enhance Memory

Lab research has shown that IF may bolster cognitive function. A study published May 2021 in Molecular Psychiatry that was performed on mice found IF was 10 percent better than traditional daily calorie restriction at enhancing long-term memory. This was an animal study, and it's unknown whether humans would experience the same results. More research is ongoing.

7. Who Shouldn't Try Intermittent Fasting, Because of Safety Concerns?

In general, health experts recommend that the following people avoid IF.

People With Type 1 Diabetes, and Those With Type 2 Who Are Taking Insulin

IF may improve insulin sensitivity, and therefore may be beneficial for people with type 2 diabetes, but it can also be risky for people on diabetes medications associated with hypoglycemia (low blood sugar), such as insulin and sulfonylureas such as glyburide, according to a study published in April 2019 in Nutrients. IF isn't recommended for people with type 1 diabetes, who rely on insulin. If you have type 2 diabetes and are curious about the diet, be sure to consult your healthcare team first.

People With Other Chronic Diseases

Not much is known about how fasting will affect many chronic diseases, including diabetes, but negative side effects such as dizziness and nausea may be more pronounced for these people, according to the 2019 Nutrients study. "You have to be careful when you have medical issues that could be worsened by not eating regularly," Lowden says. If you take medication for blood pressure or heart disease, you may be more prone to electrolyte imbalances that come with fasting, so fasting may not be recommended, per Harvard Health.

Underweight People

Those with a body mass index (BMI) of less than 18.5 are advised against any weight loss diet, including IF, according to a study published in Nutrients in March 2019.

Anyone With a History of Disordered Eating

IF may encourage an unhealthy relationship with food, according to Harvard T.H. Chan School of Public Health. A study published in June 2019 in Current Obesity Reports notes that some people may be tempted to use the end of their fast as an excuse to binge on unhealthy foods.

Elderly People

Fasting can increase the risk of cardiovascular disease, stroke, and arrhythmia among elderly people, according to the March 2019 Nutrients study.

Women Who Are Pregnant or Breastfeeding

That same study indicated that breastfeeding isn't the best time to fast or reduce calorie intake, since women need an extra 300 to 500 calories per day to keep up their energy level and milk production, according to the Mayo Clinic. Also, people who need to take medication with food should eat at regular intervals so they don't miss a dose, says Harvard Health. It's a good idea for everyone — whether you have any of the conditions listed above or not — to check with a doctor before starting a fast, per Johns Hopkins Medicine.

8. Is It Good or Bad to Exercise While Intermittent Fasting?

According to Harvard Health, one theory on the pro-exercise side is that exercising in a fasted state may make you burn fat. Lowden explains that the body needs sugar or some sort of energy to perform well while exercising.

Normally, the energy comes from sugar molecules, which are stored as glycogen in the liver. "If you start exercising, you're more likely to deplete those stores, and then your body has no choice but to go into a more anaerobic breakdown to give you the energy you need," she says. Instead of burning through sugars that aren't available, your body is forced to burn through another energy source: fat.

But you may not have enough energy to exercise as intensely as you normally would. "Peak performance or even feeling good while exercising is much easier if you eat," Lowden says.

9. What's the Best Way to Manage Hunger While Fasting?

You will likely feel hungry as your body adjusts to IF, but Gottfried says it will adjust. "From my own experience and feedback from my patients, it gets easier," she says. According to Harvard, research has found that IF doesn't increase overall appetite. Gottfried says the 16:8 diet (or some variation thereof) seems to be the easiest for most people to integrate into their lives without feeling too hungry.

10. What Side Effects Can I Expect on an Intermittent Fasting Diet?

For many people, transitioning to eating this way is not easy. Per the April 2019 Nutrients study, IF can lead to migraine, dizziness, nausea, and insomnia. It can also make people feel hungry and weak in general, limiting their activity throughout the day.

11. What Is the Best Way to Get Started on a Fasting Diet?

In addition to considering your health goals, follow these steps before diving into IF.

Talk to Your Primary Care Doctor

He or she can determine if this eating style would be beneficial for your body. "If you have questions about what is right for you, it's important to talk to healthcare professionals," Lowden says. "Everybody is an individual, and your specific doctor might have preferences about what you do and don't do based on your specific circumstances." For instance, if you often socialize late at night, 5:2 likely will be a better fit than 16:8. If you decide to try 16:8, Gottfried says to ease into it. "I recommend starting slowly at first and ramping up, with a 12-hour fast and a 12-hour eating window, then move to a 14-hour fast with a 10-hour eating window, and from there to 16:8," she says. She says to keep in mind that people have different fasting windows. "Some like to eat at 10 a.m. and stop at 6 p.m.; others prefer to wait until 12 p.m. and stop eating at 8 p.m.," she says. "Find what works for you."

Make Sure You Have Water Handy for Proper Hydration

The 2019 Nutrients study suggested drinking plenty of water during the day to reduce your risk of dehydration and to help replace fluids that you normally would source from foods.

Limit Physical Activity

It's also a good idea to limit your activities during your fasting windows until you know how your body will react, Gottfried says.

12. What Is the Best Way to Break a Fast and Begin Eating Again?

Don't take the end of your fast as an excuse to go wild with unhealthy foods — that'll undermine the potential success of the diet. "The principles of healthful eating and breaking a fast are the same whether or not it's a normal overnight fast or time-restricted eating," Lowden says. Focus on breaking your fast with a healthy, balanced meal filled with lean proteins, healthy carbohydrates, and healthy fats. Pay particular attention to protein, especially if you have diabetes. "In order [for people with diabetes] to maintain normal sugar levels and avoid worsening insulin resistance, we always recommend eating a form of protein with every meal, particularly when you're breaking a fast," Lowden says. Protein doesn't break down into glucose as efficiently as carbs, so it has a slower, less-immediate effect on blood sugar levels, according to Diabetes.co.uk.

What Midlife Women Should Know About Intermittent Fasting

Hot flashes may be the biggest challenge experienced by women around the time of menopause, but another, less-discussed concern for many are the stubborn pounds that gather around the waist and won't disappear. Some women successfully lose this extra weight when they start cutting calories or turn to a more healthful way of eating, such as the widely recommended Mediterranean diet. But other women say traditional diet plans aren't sufficient to dislodge these excess pounds in midlife — a phenomenon some have termed the "menopot." That's why many are turning to a popular eating plan known as intermittent fasting (IF).

Intermittent fasting refers to a variety of dietary schedules, all of which involve eating for a certain number of hours in a day and restricting calories in others. The method forms the cornerstone of a weight loss diet directed at menopausal women known as the Galveston diet. But the decision about whether IF is right for women over 40 needs to take into account a number of factors.

What Are the Types of Intermittent Fasting?

There are many different approaches to IF. Some people pick one to three days during the week when they eat minimally, if at all. Another technique, known as a fasting mimicking diet, severely restricts calories for five days in a month. One of the more common IF approaches recommended for weight loss involves what is called 5:2 fasting, in which you eat normally for five days in a week but seriously restrict calories, down to around 500 a day for women (600 for men), for any of the remaining two. Other people use a time restricted eating (TRE) process, eating normally during any 8 to 12 consecutive hours in a day and fasting for the remaining hours. A TRE plan that prohibits food during a 16-hour window — and leans heavily on healthy fats during the 8 hours of eating — known as 16/8, is what the Galveston diet recommends for midlife women.

What Are the Weight Loss and Health Claims of Intermittent Fasting?

The Galveston diet touts IF as a whole-health panacea in addition to a weight loss tool. According to the website, IF prevents obesity, lowers heart risks, improves insulin resistance, decreases chronic inflammation, and boosts memory, mood, and energy. Over the years, people have attributed other benefits to intermittent fasting, everything from cholesterol and blood pressure reductions to taming Alzheimer's disease and even boosting longevity.

Does the Evidence Show Intermittent Fasting Helps Midlife Women Lose Weight?

IF eating plans are not the magic bullets some tout them as online. Still, some research on intermittent fasting in adults (both men and women) has shown that they may facilitate moderate weight loss.

CONCLUSION

Intermittent fasting is a safe and sustainable way to lose weight, improve health, and adopt a healthier lifestyle. Although this method is safe to follow for most adults, it is advisable that you speak to your general practitioner before attempting intermittent fasting. This is especially important if you have underlying health conditions like diabetes, heart disease, eating disorders, low blood pressure, etc. Intermittent fasting is not recommended for women who are breastfeeding, pregnant or trying to have a baby. If you experience adverse effects while fasting or have concerns about this regimen, then do consult your doctor.